I0791045

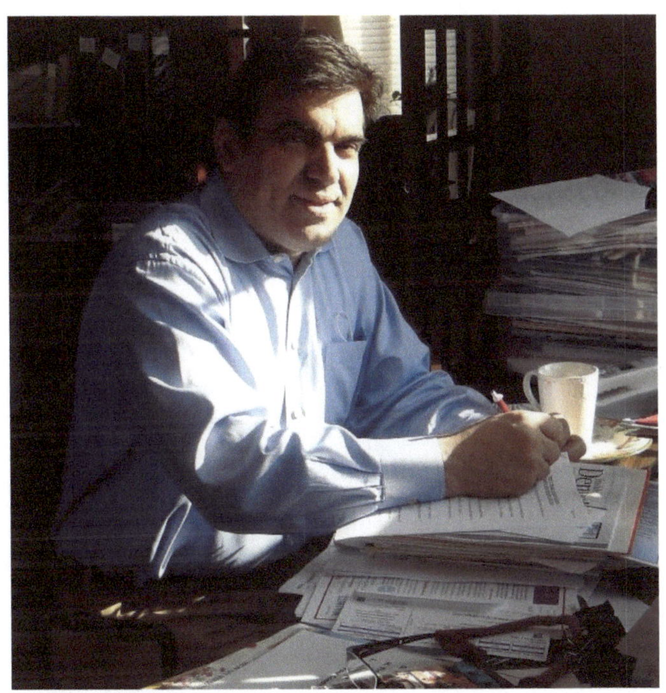

Dr. Alexander G. Alemis

Dr. Alexander G. Alemis is a dentist in Chicago, Illinois.

He has been practicing dentistry since 1986 and is the founder of

the Family Dental Care Group, a multi-group practice.

He is an accomplished businessman and author.

First Edition Copyright 2003 Alexander G. Alemis, DDS

Second Edition Copyright 2014 Alexander G. Alemis, DDS

More copies of this book can be obtained by calling

Upstat Dental Solutions at

773-978-7801

or by visiting the website

www.Dr.Alemis.com

Front Cover Art: Island of Spetses, Greece

Back Cover Art: Ermioni, Greece

ACKNOWLEDGMENTS

I would like to acknowledge many people who have helped me throughout my life. My parents, school teachers, colleagues, staff, and other friends. Nobody does it alone. Accept help, help others, and pass it on.

I would like to thank my family and my staff for putting up with my crazy schedule. A special thanks to the South Chicago Community for embracing me with open arms after graduating from dental school, as I was finding my way in the world.

Thank you!

DISCLAIMER

This book contains the thoughts and ideas of the author.
Some of the concepts presented here are abstract and
subjective and represent the opinions and experiences of
the author.

It is not intended to be a dogmatic[1] presentation nor is it
a scientific thesis[2]. It is up to the reader to agree or
disagree with the materials presented.

For any dental or other health advice and how it relates
to your overall health you need to consult your health care
provider.

---

[1] Dogmatic: to claim it's the only way and no other way
[2] Thesis: a statement or position put forth to be proven

INTRODUCTION

Many books have been written on the subject of health and its relationship to the mouth; some by dentists, some by non-dentists.

This book is different as it introduces the Subject of "Flows" and how they relate to the mouth.

The purpose of this book is to show the reader the importance the mouth and teeth play in the overall health of a person. These materials are presented in a unique manner focusing on the subject of oral health as it relates to your overall health. In the opinion of the author, **the book answers the question: "Why should I take care of my teeth?" better than any other publication around.**

To your health!

HEALTH AND FLOWS

A flow is a movement toward a certain direction.

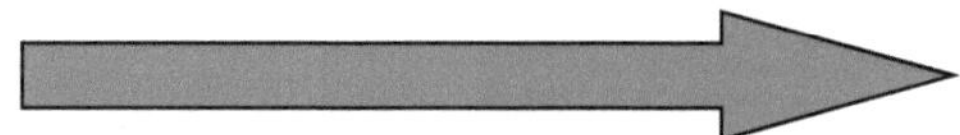

The arrow above shows movement or a flow and its direction.

A flow can be physical, such as a flow of water, air, or some other liquid.

It can also be spiritual, such as a flow of ideas, concepts, or thoughts.

Look at the following examples in pictures.

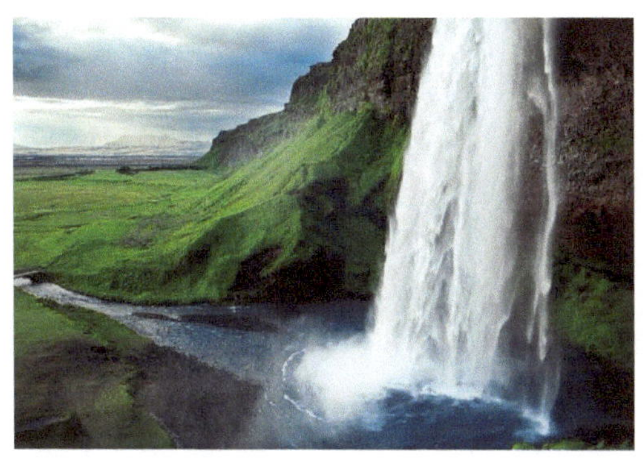

A flow of water

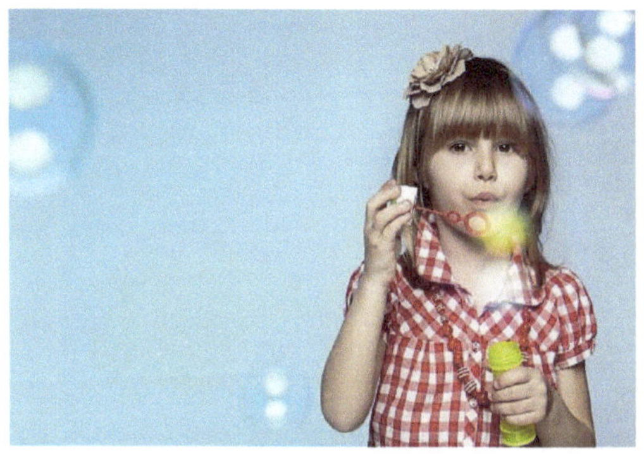

A flow of air

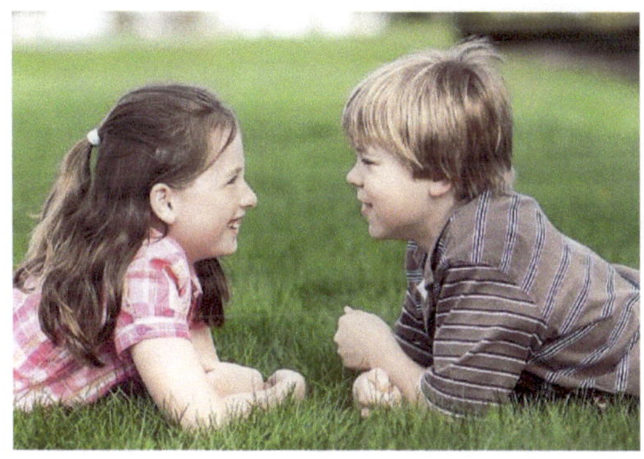

Communication: an interchange of flows

Philosophy was introduced by the ancient Greeks who studied life and wrote about it. Philosophy = Friend of Wisdom

In Greek the word "Spirit" is Pneuma, which means a flow of breath or a flow of life. The word "flow" in Greek is Roee with a long R.

By the way, since a lot of English words come from Greek most English words that have the letter "R" in them signify flows. Examples: Running, River, Row, Rhinitis[3]

An Ancient Greek philosopher used to say "ta panta ree" which means "everything flows." Life, matter, the universe, all flow as is now fully proven by physics.

So why all this background in ancient Greek philosophy and flows? What does this have to do with health?

---

[3] Rhinitis: inflammation of the nasal mucous membrane; runny nose

Apparently, the ancient Greeks felt that health was directly related to flows as the Greek word for **healthy** is **"Eurostos"** which means **good flows** and the Greek word for **"unhealthy"** is **"Arrostos"** which means **no Flows**.

Therefore, according to the ancient Greeks a person who had good flows would be healthy and one who had no flows would be sick.

Further, the Greek philosophers used to say that overall health was a combination of a healthy body and a healthy mind.

The mind, they said, affects the body and the body affects the mind.

So let's look at both. We'll look at the mind first.

MIND

A mind with good flows would be a healthy mind.

For a mind to be healthy it must be able to give and receive flows readily. It must be able to:

a. Express love, affection, and in general, feelings = Flow outwards

b. Express its own creations and accept the creation of others = Back and forth flows

c. Receive thoughts and ideas from others = Accept Inward flows

d. Receive help and help others = Back and forth flows.

All of these flows are expressed and communicated

through the mouth. So, if **healthy** is someone with **good**

flows, then if one's **flows get stuck** and one is unable to

express or receive ideas then his/her mind or spirit would

become **Arrostos = one without flows = sick.**

Now, let's look at the body.

HEALTHY BODY

The same is true about the body regarding flows. A body's healthy function is based on its ability to accept, process, and give flows.

Air with **oxygen** flows through the nose and **through the mouth** to go to the lungs. Blood flows to the lungs to pick up the oxygen and flow it throughout the tissues. **Food**, the body's nutrient, flows **through the mouth**.

The nutrients and oxygen are carried throughout the body with the flow of blood. The cells then must accept the flows of oxygen and nutrients to function. If the flow of blood stops, the body dies. In reverse, the body flows (**exhales)** the "used" air back out **through the mouth**. It must also flow out the non-processed food in terms of feces, urine, and sweat.

If at any point the flows of the body are interrupted, then the person becomes arrostos, meaning a person who has no flows = sick.

See these concepts about mind and body flows in the following diagram.

ALL FLOWS START IN THE MOUTH

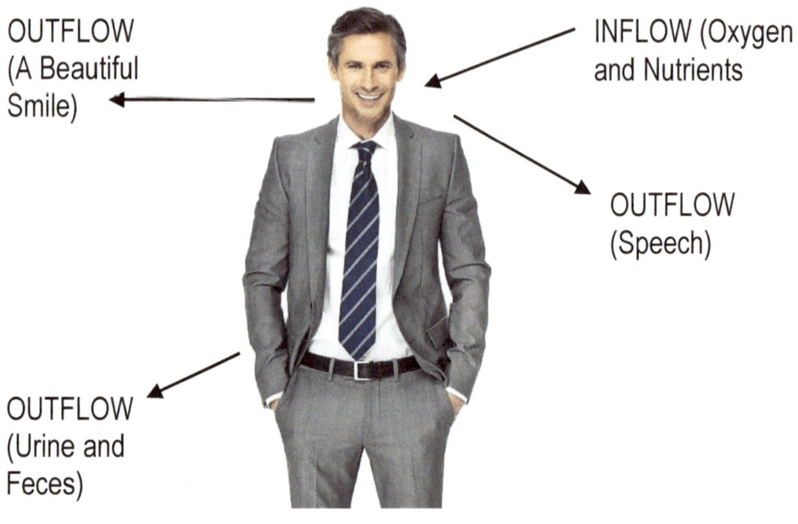

As you can see from the above, body wise **the body takes in oxygen and nutrients through the mouth** and nose and flows them through its digestive system.

Then, it flows them via the blood to the cells and discards anything unable to use through the colon, urethra, or sweat glands. Spiritually, a person communicates flows of: **ideas, concepts, thoughts, and wishes through the mouth**.

A smile is a flow in itself, the first flow people notice on another.

A beautiful smile is a good flow, a not so beautiful smile is not a good flow.

I have seen it time and again that when a person starts having problems in the **mouth, where all the flows start,** he or she begins to have problems with flows of the entire body and health deteriorates.

I believe that any kind of problem in the mouth:

A lost tooth	A sore spot
A fractured tooth	A sensitive tooth
A lost filling	An uneven bite
An infection; big or small	An ill-fitting prosthesis[4]
An infection; big or small	A worn dentition[5]

could affect our overall health, body, and mind in more ways than previously thought possible.

---

[4] Prosthesis: Replacement of a missing part of the body; in this case, an appliance to replace missing teeth
[5] Dentition: The teeth as one entity

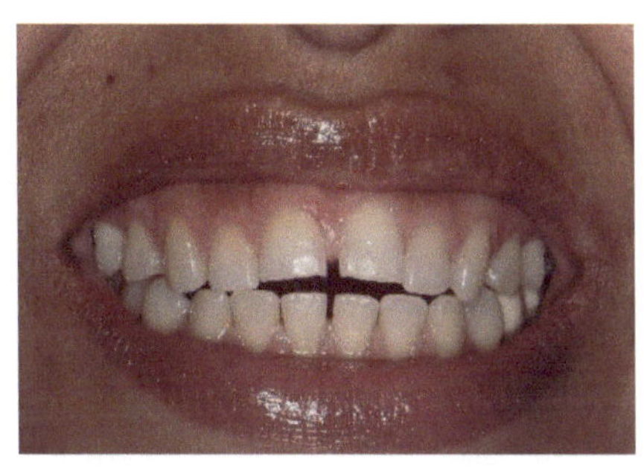

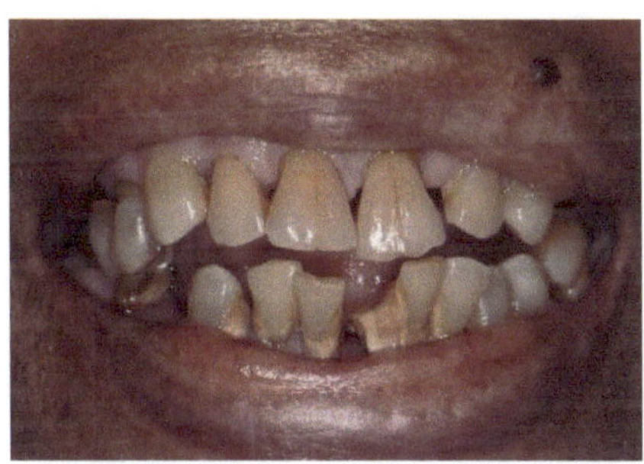

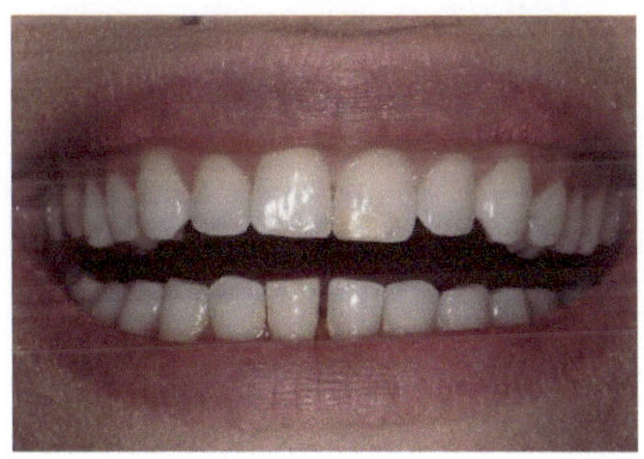

The above pictures are some examples of not good flows

It saddens me to see people who have severe health

issues such as heart condition, diabetes, or cancer and have all

sorts of problems in their oral cavity.

These patients spend hundreds of thousands of dollars

in expensive surgeries and tens of thousands of dollars on

expensive medications, yet due to problems in their oral cavity,

they cannot eat proper food to nourish their body. I even see

patients who have no teeth at all, not even dentures, yet they

have and continue to spend money and effort on all sorts of

medical treatments, in addition to drugs, to improve the health

of their body. If your body depends on what you eat to nourish

itself, then how can you sustain health if you're unable to eat

nutritional food?

On the other hand, **I have seen incredibly positive changes in the health and spirit in people who had dental issues fixed or improved.** A beautiful smile goes a long way toward feeling better about yourself and how you are perceived by others.

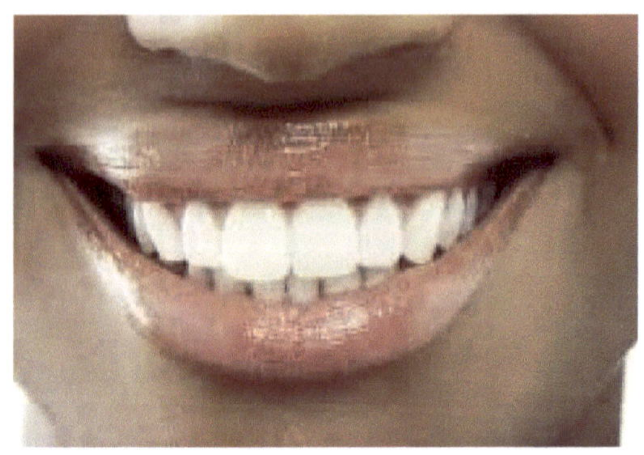

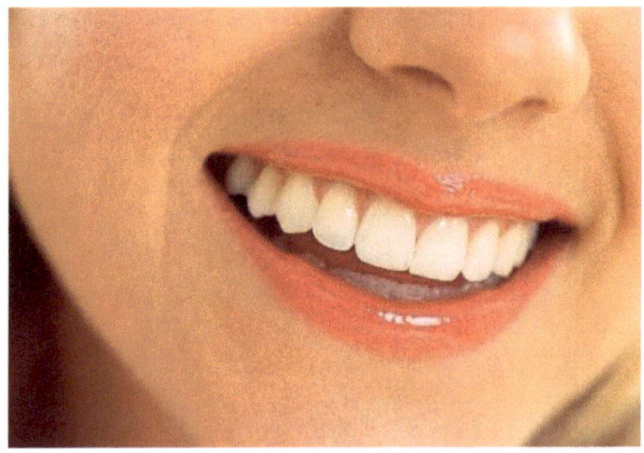

The above pictures are examples of good flows.

CONCLUSION

In order to be healthy and remain healthy, you **must**

make sure you have good flows.

      a.   Spiritually, you need to make sure others are not

            suppressing your flows

            of thoughts, ideas, or creations.

      b.   Body-wise you need to make sure you are

            breathing, eating and excreting[6] right.

If your flows become interrupted then you become

arrostos = sick.

---

[6] Excreting: eliminating waste matter from the body

All spiritual flows start in the mind and are **expressed in one form or another by the mouth.**

All body flows start in the mouth.

It's critical that the mouth has no stresses, pains, aches, or any inability to function properly. Any such problems cause an impeded[7] or stuck flow and therefore sickness begins to creep in. The first flow someone sees in you is your smile. The first positive flow you can radiate or express to the world is a beautiful smile.

BASED ON THE ABOVE, I BELIEVE IT IS CRITICAL THAT ANY PROBLEMS IN THE MOUTH BE FIXED AS SOON AS POSSIBLE BECAUSE THE MOUTH PLAYS SUCH A CRITICAL ROLE IN EVERYONE'S HEALTH.

---

[7] Impeded: slowed down or stopped

Other Works by the Author

Intelligence: How Intelligent are you? Discover the 63 Traits of Intelligence: This book breaks intelligence down into 63 distinct traits, some innate, and others that can be acquired by learning about them. Can you increase your intelligence and thereby your ability to solve life's problems and capitalize on opportunities presented in life?

Political Systems and Their Relationship to the Economy and Freedom: A simple yet powerful work on understanding how different political systems affect the economy and how the free enterprise system is the most proven system to create prosperity for people.

Hellenism: Freedom on Earth: An interesting insight on the roots of Western Civilization.

Things to Do Daily Notebook: A powerful tool to assist with your daily schedule.

UDS Dental Management Technology: This consists of ten volumes of approximately 3000 pages of a comprehensive management system and several seminars on how to run a dental office.

Task Management System: A software program to help executives better assign and monitor assigned tasks.

17 Rules or Rules to Fix Any Economy Anywhere in the World: People make the economy. They are similar, regardless of color, culture or creed, but they are shaped by the systems or rules they live under. Change the rules to change the economy, if that is what you desire of course.

www.ingramcontent.com/pod-product-compliance
Lightning Source LLC
Chambersburg PA
CBHW040252240726
48664CB00001B/366